Lose The Weight

Losing Weight Naturally, Weight Loss Motivation, Fitness Diet & Mindset

99 Weight Loss Tips

By: Amy Culderson and Mike Shaw

Amy Culderson and Mike Shaw

LOSE THE WEIGHT PREFACE:

Congratulations for taking a big step in your weight loss journey. The start is always the toughest part, and because you purchased this book, you are showing yourself that you want to lose weight, and you are going to do what it takes to lose it!

This book is broken up into 5 different sections: The Start, Motivation & Mindset, On The Daily, Diet & Food, and Fitness & Exercise. All of the tips in this book are completely natural ways of losing the weight and keeping it off, so you can be assured that you are not only losing weight, but staying healthy while doing it.

Take the tips that we've learned over many years of fitness, diet, and most recently motivation and mindset. Enjoy the tips, use your favorites starting today, stick to them, and watch your success.

Main Sections:

The Start

Motivation/Mindset

On The Daily

Diet & Food

Fitness/Exercise

Bonus Section: Immediate Results!

THE START OF YOUR WEIGHT LOSS JOURNEY

Everyone starts somewhere, and even if you think your weight problem can't be solved, these tips should get you going in the right direction so that you don't have to worry about any form or type of surgery, crazy pills or no-food diets.

Before you hop on a treadmill or stop eating large meals, you must first have the mindset, the plan, and the goal(s). Without a clear mindset and end goal in mind, your road to losing weight will be rocky, full of obstacles, and might lead you down some alternate routes.

In this very first tip, we'll go over briefly how to make a plan and set up goals for yourself so that you always have something to look forward to. Right after making your plan, we'll dive right into motivation and mindset, where you will continue to program your mind and body to be healthier, and to get in the right state of mind to be able to tackle the task of losing weight for good.

1

MAKE A PLAN, SET GOALS

Without a plan, you're toast. What, are you just going to get on the treadmill and just start running? Although it seems like a good plan, most will falter away from running without a clear plan and goals. Non-planning is for the people who end up quitting one week (or worse, one day) in.

To make a plan, just start with something you could see yourself doing every day for a year. Don't plan on running a mile every day. But maybe you could walk around the block, or maybe do some elastic-band exercises every morning. Starting with something small makes it easy to do it over and over. Eventually you'll want to challenge yourself more instead of being beat to death from the start.

After making your initial plan, it is important to set some goals as well. Maybe you want to lose 30 pounds, maybe you want to just be that size 6 or 4 or whatever again. Whatever it is, set that goal, and make it difficult as well as obtainable. You want to be able to reach this goal without going crazy. You can always pass up your goal and set new ones later ;)

With a solid plan and goals, you are many steps ahead of the others trying to lose weight.

Motivation, Mindset and More

Section 2 of this book is all about motivation and mindset.

You now have a plan and some goals set up, but what happens if you procrastinate? What happens if you just stop alltogether?

These tips will help you clear our mind and fill it with motivation to get you going again in no time.

2

LIST OF DISADVANTAGES

Sure you know the advantages of losing weight: look better, feel better, able to do more, more energized, more attractive, healthier on the inside, less risk for disease (and countless more).

But sometimes we can't get motivated simply because the advantages are already known, meaning they are obtainable at another time in the future (literally whenever we want). If you know you can start to lose 20 pounds a month or two from now, it's easy to say you'll wait. But if you know and say to yourself that you are more at risk for disease, or that you are out of breath just walking around the mall - those disadvantages of not losing weight can outweigh the advantage of losing it.

This is how a lot of previous smokers quit smoking. Instead of attaching the positive vibe of feeling healthier, they attach the negative vibe of not dying from lung cancer. Now, I wouldn't recommend always pointing to the negative energy, but you can see that you can use negative energy and thoughts and turn them into motivation to do what needs to be done. When you then start working on losing weight, the positive energy will come.

3

MOTIVATING YOURSELF

Sometimes, there's no one out there that understands. No one you can talk to. I understand, I've been there before.

When it seems like there's no one there, no one you can talk to, you need to find ways of motivating yourself. Like the previous tip of listing disadvantages of not losing the weight, you must put together some sort of verbal, mental, or visual cue that gets you back into that specific mindset of wanting to lose weight.

It can be as easy as saying some positive things to yourself over and over. You could meditate for 10 minutes, or listen to some music. I like to close my eyes and think about what I will look like in the future after I put in the work. Just block out everything and everyone else, and give yourself the mental image of your future, thinner, healthier self.

Then open your eyes, and get back to work! Right now it might seem difficult to understand how to just motivate yourself out of thin air, but when you use some of the later tips in this book, you will attach those tips, techniques, diets, exercises, mental images etc. to your motivation tactics, and you won't have much of a problem motivating yourself because you'll have so many things to choose from.

4

MAINTAIN PROPER POSTURE

This is a fun quick tip that many people have heard a million times, but might not know that it can help you lose weight.

Do you find that you are slouching a lot?

When you sit down, is your butt up against the back of the seat where it meets the back part? When you walk, do you hold your head up with your neck and walk strong or does your head sort of sink into your neck and is held up by your shoulders?

These are all questions to ask yourself, because they can really help with losing weight. If you walk slowly and hardly move your arms and your head is only being held up by your shoulders, that's a problem. Walk with a purpose, move your arms back and forth when you walk, hold your head up high. Don't turn your full body to look to the left and right, turn your head.

When you have correct posture and really pay attention to the tiny things you do (or don't do) all day, it helps immensely with losing weight. Remember, it's the little things that count. I'm not saying this will "shave off a pound a week" or anything - all I'm saying is it helps with the big picture. Feeling better, thinking better thoughts, planning, getting motivated, exercising, doing little things during the day.

Proper posture is just one of those little things that helps, so start to pay attention to it starting now.

5

INFORM FAMILY OF PLANS

If you want to lose weight faster than ever before, tell your family about it.

Tell your sibling(s) and parent(s) that you have a plan to lose weight, and that you will be working hard to achieve a specific goal.

When you tell your family about your weight loss plan, it's easier to get support when you are procrastinating or feeling unmotivated. Maybe one of your family members will make fun of you. Maybe one won't support you at all. Maybe another will support you too much to the fact where they are overbearing and almost forceful with your plan.

Family is family. If you know you won't get support from one person or another, there's always extended family, friends, school mates and more. Letting your friends and family know of your plan to lose weight will allow them to make some minor adjustments in their daily life. Maybe your mom or husband or wife or whoever won't make you dinners with lots of saturated fat or salt or meat. Maybe your brother or sister or friend won't ask to get ice cream every day. Maybe you'll inspire someone else to do a fun physical activity with you each week!

You never know until you try. Inform others of your plans and keep going.

6

DREAM ABOUT LOSING WEIGHT (ENVISION)

Earlier in the book, I told you about my technique involving closing my eyes and envisioning myself skinny. This is similar.

In order to really lose the weight and keep it off, you must dream about it, you must envision it as if it has already happened. Put your future skinny self in front of a thousand people. Look at the way they look at you. You are accomplished, you are healthy, skinny, you feel great, you look great.

Envision yourself walking into the doctor's office for a physical, and getting the test results back saying you are as healthy as someone can be. Envision getting on a rollercoaster and being able to hear more than 2 clicks when you pull down the support rail.

When you have a clear dream of not only how you will look, but also of how life will be like for you, it helps you stay in that mindset, and you will attract your thoughts and dreams into your life.

7

Picture Prior

This is an easy tip and although you see it online and in weight loss ads, there are many people that don't do this but should!

I call it "Picture Prior", and it's basically a picture of yourself prior to losing weight. Take a picture of yourself right now, full body, and save that picture, keep it close by.

A month from now, take another picture. Keep taking pictures, and keep tracking your success. When you can see your face change shape within a few weeks to a few months, it makes it that much more worth it to keep going. Besides, you wouldn't want to go back to what you were like at picture #1, would you?

8

WEIGHT LOSS COMPETITION

I've seen both guys and girls do personal weight loss competitions with eachother. And when I say competition, I don't mean "Biggest Loser" or any widely known network shows.

I'm talking about the weight loss competition (or "BET") you have with friends to see who can lose 10 pounds the quickest, who can lose the most in a month, and similar bets like that.

When you can get more of your friends and family involved, it makes it fun. A little competition is always healthy. AND - what makes this even more worthwhile is if you add a WAGER. Winner gets $100 from the others? Losers have to buy winner a vacation?

Put in a wager, run a little weight loss competition, and you'll be more motivated than ever.

9

GET YOURSELF A DOG

If you want something that will force you to lose some weight and get moving, GET YOURSELF A DOG!!

You thought I'd title the chapter "get yourself a dog" and be joking with you? I'm serious, getting a dog could be the best thing that ever happened to you. And I'm not talking about having a family dog that someone else takes care of. If you own a dog and don't walk it or do much of the taking care of, then this tip might not work for you (same goes if you aren't a dog person).

When you have a dog that you love and care for, it will keep you motivated and ready to do something. Besides walking the dog, just playing with a frisbee or ball outside, or even the act of going out and getting dog food, opening up the package, filling it up once or twice a day - it all gets you moving.

Your best bet is to do a little research on different types of dogs. There are some breeds of dogs that can work with your own lifestyle, so instead of having to go on 3 long fast-paced walks a day, some dogs only require getting outside and running around the yard while you play fetch or other games with your dog.

All in all, a dog gets you moving, and the more you're in motion, the easier it is to lose weight - remember that.

10

WATCH SPORTS ON TV

Your worst enemy is the Food Network or similar food channel on TV. I'll agree that sometimes they have some healthy delicious food on their shows, but it's seeing people eating in general that makes us want to eat as well.

Try watching sports. Trust me, even if you aren't a sports fanatic, there are still many different sports to choose from, and you don't even have to watch any particular game or understand every rule. I understand most sports, and although I don't understand hockey, I'll watch it when it comes on. It gets me subconsciously pumped up.

Just like any other mindset and motivation technique, it's all about what you think about and what you envision that starts the motivation, the feeling, the action to do something. Watch sports every once in awhile. Think about how hard a person had to work to get to where they are. If they can do that, there's no doubt that you can lose a few pounds.

And hey, you might even find a new favorite sport to watch, or better yet, try!

11

GET OTHERS INVOLVED

Just like before when I told you about starting a competition with friends, it's really inspiring to get more people involved in one common goal.

You can do a competition or bet, but sometimes it's nice to just work with others to keep eachother motivated. When it's just you, it can get tough to push yourself to exercise one day, or hold back on the greasy fries. But when friends and family are involved in the same goal, you can keep eachother on track.

It's also nice to get others involved, because when one person tries to comfort another person who might have stopped exercising, it feels more like comfort rather than nagging someone, because they are right there with you going through the same thing. It's harder to get told, "Go do this on your own" rather than "come do this with me" or "let me do this with you".

12

CONSIDER YOUR BODY'S NEEDS

Just like we have emotional needs, our body has physical needs as well.

It might feel really really good to bite into a cheeseburger, and will make our emotions turn happy and satisfied. However, what might feel good at first is really damaging the inside and outside of your body little by little. Each time you eat acidic or fatty, greasy foods, you are damaging your body.

When I was overweight, some people who I really loved would tell me I needed to lose weight, get healthier. I hated them at first, I thought they were making fun of me - I thought, "I'm fine the way I am". But when my doctor told me I was at risk for Diabetes, I realized my family was not trying to hurt my emotional being. They were trying to help my physical being.

Although I believe you look beautiful just the way you are, this thing we call life tells us that it will last longer if we live healthier. Take some time to consider the needs of your body - think of your physical body like a car. You put in bad oil, and get bad production. Parts get gunky, pieces come apart. One part gets damaged, eventually it hurts another part. Before you know it, the engine is completely fried. But unlike a car, you can't replace a human life.

13

MAKING WEIGHT LOSS
INTERESTING

We all love playing games, so why not make weight loss fun by making a game out of it?

You can make weight loss interesting in a whole lot of different ways, you just have to get creative. You could reward yourself by seeing a new movie every time you lose weight each week.

Besides rewards, try beating your weight loss goals each week from the week previous. If you lost 2 pounds last week, try losing 3 this week. Then next week lose 4 or 5! It's okay if you lose a game or don't complete your goal tasks right away or all the time. The point is making weight loss fun to keep you going.

14

MONITOR/JOURNAL YOUR WEIGHT LOSS

This is something every weight loser must do. I know, I know, it's hard to keep tracking your weight because sometimes it fluctuates all over the place! That's okay... If you gain a pound or two, it's not the end of the world.

However, although it's not the end of the world to gain weight, it's important that you track and journal your weight loss so that you can cut out bad habits or change up your routine to accomplish your goals.

Not only should you be monitoring your weight in pounds (or kilograms) each week, but you should also be journaling daily or at least bi-weekly about what you eat, what you do during the day - any big meals you had, etc. When you can track these things, it makes it much easier to find out why you might have gained some weight one week and lost a lot another. And when you find a few weeks that are BIG losers, take a look at your journal for those weeks and find out what you did to lose the weight, and keep doing that!

15

REWARDING YOURSELF

If you can't think of any weight loss games or alternative ways of making weight loss interesting, you can always go with the tried and true reward system.

Mark out your goals - "I want to lose 10 pounds in one month."

Then, tell yourself what reward you will give yourself when you have completed that goal - "I will go to the spa" or "I will go to the sports game" or any other reward.

It's best to stay away from food-related goals as much as you can, unless of course you are rewarding yourself for a larger goal like half of your entire goal weight lost. You don't want to reward yourself with a cheeseburger and milkshake for every pound you lose, or you'll be losing one and gaining 3 each week. But if you wanted to lose 20 pounds and lost 10 so far, you can make a food-related reward.

When you can see the end reward and result, it is easier to make it happen.

16

GROCERY STORE ONLY AFTER...

Take a visit to the grocery store, but only after eating first!

Think about it: You're hungry. You haven't eaten all day. You go to the grocery store. While looking around, you see foods that will fill you up - meat, snacks, chips, ice cream, cookies, candy, and more. Salad? Haha, that's not going to make this tummy rumblin' go away!

See what I mean? You can't go to grocery store hungry expecting to come out with healthy food. And once you've bought your unhealthy food and bring it home, you've only wasted your money on food that is going to add excess pounds onto your body and make you more unhealthy.

So, make sure you eat a full meal before you go the grocery store. Whether it is breakfast lunch or dinner, just make sure you have a full stomach. You'll find that while browsing throughout the grocery aisles, you will have more conscious thoughts about your food choices instead of your subconscious need for energy or simply something to fill you up.

17

VACATION WORKOUT PLAN

Working out on vacation? Hell yeah, why not?

I'm not saying you have to run a marathon. But you'll find that most vacation places have some sort of gym or workout area - and some are quite nice.

If you are going to a nice hotel or on a cruise, take advantage of the high quality beautifully workout equipment they have. Many resorts will have saunas and hot tubs and steam rooms. You'd think working out on vacation would be a burden, but it can in fact be relaxing and enjoyable.

If you are traveling somewhere that might not have a workout area or gym in the facility or close by, there are always little things you can do while on vacation that will keep your weight loss goals intact. Try taking a walk around the area. Use the stairs more than the elevator.

When you first wake up in the morning before everyone else, do some stretching and leg and arm exercises in your room. Take a swim if it's nice out.

I always try to plan out some sort of physical activity during my vacations, even if the activity seems small or unimportant. To be completely honest, working out during vacation gives me way more energy than the people I go with. You'd think that the person who sleeps 12 hours would be well rested and ready to have a full day, right? Wrong. Even after 12 hours of sleep, they take another hour to really wake up, another hour to get situated and ready to go, then they are hungry, then they want to relax and sit again, then it's almost time for dinner. But me on the other hand - I'll wake up at 7am after 8 or 9 hours of sleep, work out for an hour (easy/medium workout), and be pumped and ready to do anything for the rest of the day. It allows me to do more things and have more fun while I'm on vacation.

18

DON'T BE TOO
HARD ON YOURSELF

Like I've said before, it's okay if you gain weight some weeks. Don't be too hard on yourself.

No one is perfect - not me, not you, not anyone. If you gain 5 pounds this week, that's okay, it's not the end of the world. Instead of being hard on yourself, start to look at situations from a bird's eye view and you'll find that they aren't hard to change.

So you gained 5 pounds. Let's take a step back - Did you eat a lot one day? How often did you exercise? Have you been thinking negatively lately?

Instead of being problem oriented, be solution oriented. Don't beat the problem over and over or it will become a bigger problem. Find a solution (or just one of many) and run with it. You will be less hard on yourself and more successful in your weight loss plan when you can focus on solutions more than problems.

19

FIND A PARTNER FOR SUCCESS

You've learned that it's both inspirational and fun to get others involved in your weight loss goals.

But having that one person that is basically your right hand partner in your weight loss journey can be even more inspiring. You can keep others involved as well, but it's great to have that one person you can go to and talk to and work out with when you need motivation.

My mother didn't need to lose weight, but was having problems with her back and her hips, and the doctor recommended her working out a few times a week. She couldn't stick to a plan until she got her best friend involved. Her best friend can't work out as much or as hard, but is recovering from surgery on her knees and was also recommended light work outs with specific exercises.

So, my mom and her best friend became workout partners, and more-so eachother's accountability partners. When one was too tired or not interested, the other would say, "Come on, you know it's fun when we're down there. You don't have to work out hard, let's just go for a little bit." And they go, they have a great time, and as soon as they are there they forget about any other notion about working out beforehand.

Get a partner that will motivate you and keep you going, and make sure you do the same for them!

20

SET SHORT TERM GOALS

Having trouble losing 100 pounds? Well when you think about just how heavy 100 pounds is, I would have trouble losing it too.

But what about losing 20 pounds? Sounds a little easier. 10 pounds doesn't seem that hard when we were just talking about 100. Let's break it down even further to just 5 pounds.

If you want to SEE the results and really show and track that you are hitting your goals and completing tasks, try setting some shorter-term goals. If you are 180 pounds and want to be 120, then break your 60-pound weight loss journey down into 12 sections of 5 pounds each. Make your short term goals losing that NEXT 5 pounds.

When you have checked off a few short term goals, you can set bigger ones. Maybe instead of just losing 5 or 10 pounds at a time, you want to lose 10 pounds by a specific date. Then you can track it by day to make sure you hit that 10 pound goal.

It feels nice to check something off the list, and I think because we as humans love accomplishing things. We'd rather accomplish losing 1 pound 60 times rather than losing 60 pounds 1 time. So set up some short term goals now, and reach the first one within the next few days.

21

LATE NIGHTS = BAD NEWS

The dreaded late night...

Look, late nights can be fun, entertaining, maybe even peaceful. However, late nights can also lead to bad physical and mental habits that can affect your weight loss journey.

The later you stay up, the harder it is to get up in the morning, the harder it is to get motivated to do anything productive. The later you stay up, the more you have the tendency to eat and drink. And not only are you adding on extra weight to your body while you are up during these late hours, but then all of the food sits in your stomach while you sleep. This stretches your stomach for the next day, making you feel more hungry, making you eat more food.

There's a whole lot of crap that comes with late nights, so try avoiding them as much as possible unless you know that you are able to control your thoughts and your actions, both during the late night and the next morning.

22

PRIOR DOCTOR VISIT

Before going on a weight loss journey, it's smart to visit your doctor for a quick checkup or physical.

Have your doctor run tests for body fat, have them do a full physical and ask them questions about your health and that you want to lose weight. They will tell you where you are at physically right now, and can tell you if there is anything wrong with you or anything to look out for before starting with your exercising, diets, and changes.

If you are doing a thorough checkup as most do, you should be given charts and sheets with lots of numbers, maybe some graphs and percentages. Keep this handy, as you will want to visit the doctor after you have reached your weight loss goals (and probably during as well). Not only will you be able to see your progress right in front of you, but you will also be notified if there is anything wrong with you that might prevent you from doing a specific diet or exercise.

23

READ WEIGHT LOSS
SUCCESS STORIES

Don't be bitter about other people's success. So many people hate the people who they want to look like, be like, have as much as. But when you have a hate or bitterness or jealousy towards people, you are putting the negative thoughts in your head that those people are bad, or that you shouldn't be like those people.

So when you look at weight loss success stories, don't immediately say, "Well screw this person, they look great and I can never look that good!". Instead, look at the success and say "This person found out how to lose the weight, and I'm finding out how right now as well."

Read the success stories as if you are scheduled to be the next one. Pretend that you have a deadline coming up, and it needs to be YOUR weight loss success story. If you had a deadline for work or school, you'd get it in on time, right? Same goes for weight loss. Be that next success story. Read them all, see what they have in common. Hard work, persistence, daily action, mindset, exercise, eating smaller portions more frequently - you'll probably find other common stories as well.

If you want to make a lot of money, take advice from someone who's made a lot, not from someone who is broke. If you want to lose weight, take advice from someone who has lost a lot, not from someone who hasn't been in that position before. Learn how others obtained success, then obtain it for yourself in the same way.

24

LOSING WEIGHT IN
A HEALTHY WAY

I stated this briefly in the preface of this book, but I wanted to reiterate this to make it clear: Make absolutely sure that you are losing weight in a healthy way.

Trust me, I've seen too many problems, drama and disasters with unnatural pills, life-threatening diets, surgeries, and more.

Some weight losers have trouble losing weight for awhile. It's not a huge problem until they are told they could die if they gain any more weight. All of a sudden, because they believe losing weight is hard, that they should go through surgery or take pills or just stop eating all together.

They believe pills, diets, and surgeries are the only way out, as if the problems that can occur are better than the problems that can occur from being overweight. The problem is, their lives can become even more unhealthy once the weight is lost using unnatural techniques. Surgery leaves scars for life and sometimes surgery fails later in life or needs to be redone. Pills can cause problems such as addition, or other diseases and eating disorders (not to mention can really cause damage to your insides). Dieting is okay until it is taken too far - eating nothing for days is not a good idea, and can cause many problems if not death.

The best way to lose weight is the natural way, no doubt. I just wanted to say it again so you know that I'm looking out for you. Don't worry about the models and celebrities and doctors telling you that you need their product in order to look thin, beautiful, wanted. You can lose weight naturally and quietly laugh at those people telling you otherwise.

25

STAYING ACTIVE (CONTINUE)

This can be a fun game, or can be more of a daily mission. I call it CONTINUE.

Basically, as soon as you wake up, you are to continue doing things all day long. Not once should you be sitting around doing nothing, wondering what to do.

Start by waking up and immediately stretching. While you are stretching, plan out your day. There are obviously things you have to do - maybe school, work, drop off kids, get dropped off somewhere, who knows - but there are things you NEED to do. Besides those things, think about other things you can do in between the main daily tasks.

Before work or school you could make a healthy breakfast. Walk the dog maybe? Take a walk around the block if you have 15 extra minutes. After school or work you can organize the house a little, clean maybe, learn something new, read a book, take another walk.

Just keep doing things all day long - that's the mission. When you program your mind and your daily action part of your brain to always want to do things and stay motivated, you will find that in the future, as soon as you sit down and get even an ounce of boredom, something will hit you saying "What else can I do right now?"

26

WATCH TV ONLY AFTER...

This goes along with your "CONTINUE" mission that we covered in the previous weight loss tip.

You want to be doing things all day. What isn't involved in the "things" is watching TV. However, we all know that there are things we just love to do. Maybe it's gaming, computer browsing, internet surfing, TV watching, movie watching. They aren't the most productive, but they aren't detrimental to your health in small doses.

Instead of allowing yourself to watch TV whenever you want, try watching TV or doing your 'fun' activity only after you have done everything else you needed to do, including working out, exercising, stretching, or something active.

When you can hold back your rewards, even if they are as small as watching TV, you will become more persistent in your efforts to not only lose weight but also in your life in general.

27

DON'T WORK WHERE YOU EAT

Do you do busy work (or worse, work from your job or business) in the kitchen or at the dining room table?

Bad idea if you want to lose weight.

When you work or remain in an area that has a lot of food or a place where you eat frequently, you tend to want to snack on something or nibble on something. This is because your mind is remembering that you are in an area that you have eaten food in the past, so your mind tells your stomach it's time to eat.

If you work at home or if you just browse on the computer at home, it's best to do it in your bedroom, office, or some place where you don't frequently eat food or store food. You will have less cravings for food or snacks, and will program your mind to wait on eating until you are actually hungry. You don't want to starve yourself, but you definitely don't want to overeat due to boredom or little mind tricks like working where you eat.

Besides not working where you eat, start looking at your surroundings and think about what you can do to get yourself more energized and less bored.

28

BUY SMALLER CLOTHES

"There's nothing worse than being too big to fit into my own clothes," she says.

It's even worse when you are the one spending the money on the clothes. But besides the disappointed feeling it gives you, not fitting into your clothes can actually motivate you more than you think.

My brother was starting to get a little gut, and then one year it got really bad. He had gained 40 pounds almost in months, and it was only when we talked one day that we found out how it happened (or at least one of the reasons). Instead of buying clothes that fit him, he would get the elastic clothing, one-size-fits-all clothing, stuff that breathes.

At the moment, he thought he was taking the pressure off of his belly and body by buying and wearing looser clothes. However, although he was more comfortable for the time being, he had prepared for his belly to get bigger, and had told his subconscious mind to gain weight so that he could fit into these loose clothes.

I told him to try buying smaller clothes, and after a little arguing he decided to try it. He bought a few jeans a couple sizes too small. He would try to put them on but couldn't. However, something happened over those next few weeks. His mindset changed (slowly but surely), and in a couple weeks he was able to fit into some smaller clothes. When he did it a second time, he decided to go all out. He bought pants and shirts at the size he wanted to fit in after his entire gut was gone, and was able to achieve that goal in less than a year.

It might not work for everyone, but you might want to give it a shot, just try it out and see if anything changes. It all starts in the mind.

29

DONATE YOUR LARGER CLOTHES

On top of buying smaller clothes to motivate yourself to lose weight quicker, you should also donate all of your larger clothes to Goodwill, any homeless shelter, friends and family. Just get rid of them.

If you want to fit in that dress, or that suit, or those shirts and pants, you can't expect to do it while still owning your larger clothes. I'm not saying to get rid of all the clothes that may be large but still fit you. But heck, get rid of most of them.

When you donate your larger clothes, you are telling the world and yourself that you are done with being this big, and you don't need these clothes because you'll never be that big to fit in them ever again anyway. They are worthless to you, because you are only going to get smaller.

And that's why buying smaller clothes at the same time helps out a lot with donating your larger clothes, because not only do you get to rid yourself of the big clothes, you also don't fall under the trap of telling yourself that you "have nothing to wear". Instead, you'll know you have something to wear, but you just need to lose some more weight in order for it to fit.

30

GET ENOUGH SLEEP

Sleep energizes you, gets you ready for the day ahead. Without it, you get lethargic, lazy, bored, tired. Without enough sleep, your day becomes instantly unproductive.

In a previous weight loss tip I told you to wake up an hour earlier. Well if you're currently only getting 5 hours of sleep, you definitely shouldn't take that tip. In fact, you should be getting more sleep.

Oversleeping is bad, undersleeping is worse. You get less done, you become more stressed, more irritable. With stress comes eating, then overeating. You become sad, depressed, eat more. Then you stay up late and get even less sleep. It's a vicious cycle that can be stopped at the root.

Just get enough sleep. Get yourself energized and ready for the day. If you need a nap, take a 30 minute nap during the day. Just don't turn that nap into 3 hours of TV shows.

31

RELIEVE YOUR STRESS

Stress can be caused by many things other than not sleeping enough.

If you feel stressed more often than not, it's very important that you take some time during the day to relax and relieve your stress. It can be as simple as doing some breathing exercises or counting to 10, or more involved like silent meditation or boxing.

Next time you are stressed, try relieving your stress, and once it is relieved, take note of what helped so you can use that stress reliever technique next time you need it.

The reason you want to relieve your stress is because stress is one of those things in life that can cause dozens of other outcomes. Stress can cause depression, and depression can cause overeating. Stress can also lead to overeating on it's own, can upset your stomach and lead to even more serious problems.

If you want to lose weight, keeping the stress at a minimum is a good start. If you are happy, it's easier to get healthy.

32

BE ACTIVE AT PARTIES

This tip is for you party-goers.

Be active at parties. Don't be the lazy guy or girl that sits on the couch drinking and/ or eating all night long. Get up, walk around to different people instead of letting them come to you.

Put simply, when you are more active at parties, you burn more carbs as well as keep yourself ready enough to wake up the next day. I'm not saying to not have a good time at parties, but don't get so plastered that you are going to sleep for 14 hours into the next day's afternoon. And don't sit down the entire time eating or drinking alcohol either. Alcohol just adds onto the belly, so pace yourself.

As you might notice, it's all about finding that happy medium to keep your weight loss goals on track. Doing nothing won't help you lose weight, but taking 5 pills a day and only eating lemons for a week isn't safe at all. Most people expect to lose weight from some 1 magic miracle, whether it's a potion or lotion, or spell or pill or injection or surgery. But, the truth of the matter is that weight loss can be easily achieved simply by doing the little things.

We've written this book for you so that instead of focusing your energy on a super workout routine or only drinking some magic drink for food, you can instead enjoy losing weight by just following some simple tips and changing a few things in your life. Not overdoing it at parties or any gathering for that matter (even by yourself) is one of them.

33

WEIGHT LOSS BAG VISUALIZATION

I absolutely love this and recommend it for EVERYONE on a weight loss journey! Yes, it's that inspiring.

This is called weight loss bag visualization, and involves you actually seeing and feeling the weight that you lose.

You can do this in a variety of ways, but the easiest is using a strong sack of some sort and sand (you can also use rocks, dirt, garbage, anything really). You might also want a little bit of string or a stretch cord to wrap the top closed.

So week 1 you lose 5 pounds. So, you take 5 pounds of sand, dirt, or whatever you want, and pour it into the empty sack. Pick it up, feel the weight that you've taken off yourself. Do this each week. A month from now, you might have 5, 10, 20 or more pounds in that sack. As the months go on, the sack will get heavier and heavier, further solidifying your goal of losing all the weight.

During your weight loss journey, you can also do some motivational exercises with the sack of lost weight. When your bag is 20 pounds heavy, try carrying it on your back for an hour. Try attaching it to your belly and see if you can walk with that thing! I cried when I couldn't even pick up my sack of lost weight. I thought to myself, "How on earth could I have carried all this weight for this long?"

This is truly an eye opener for everyone I do this with, and I want you to be next.

34

Your "Future Advantage" List

We've talked about using negative energy as positive energy, we've even talked about simple tricks to motivating yourself to lose the weight.

This is called the "future advantage" list, where you will list all the things you will do and have a new advantage on when all the weight is gone.

Get out a piece of paper and a pen, or open up a document on the computer, and get going on this fun exercise. What will you do when you are your perfect body weight? Have you wanted to go rock climbing or hiking? Maybe ride that roller coaster you couldn't fit on a year ago?

You can even write down how others will view you when you are thinner. It's a fact that you will be taken more seriously, either consciously or subconsciously, because people will have the vision of you taking care of yourself, meaning you can probably take care of other people, or are more motivated, or are perceived to be able to get bigger or more involved jobs or tasks done.

List all of your future advantages, and glance at them every day. The more weight you lose, the more real these advantages become.

35

SEE YOURSELF SKINNY

Have you ever wanted to actually see yourself skinny?

Well, in today's technological world, you can now actually see yourself skinny using free online websites and applications.

I won't list any specific apps or sites as they change all the time, but I'm telling you about them because these little sites and apps as a whole aren't going anywhere - people love them and use them too much.

Essentially, you upload a picture of yourself into their app using their easy instructions (basically just centering yourself into their head/body frame), and in seconds your image is altered to a view of you skinny.

This could actually be the best little weight loss tool out there, because instead of envisioning in your mind or using bags of sand, you can actually SEE yourself as you want to look in the near future.

So go ahead, find some of these sites and apps, upload your picture, get your skinny-fied image, and print that baby out. Post it to your wall, your door, next to your computer, put it in your wallet or purse. Envision yourself skinny, and your thoughts and actions will begin to change for the better.

WEIGHT LOSS IN YOUR DAILY ROUTINE

Section 3 is all about weight loss in your daily routine. We felt like including this little section of a few daily routine tips would help the overall audience that we are going for.

Everyone has a daily routine, whether or not we admit it. We can't all live like rockstars (and even they have routines!). We all have tasks or jobs or hobbies or things we do during the day, and there are a few things you can do in order to help you lose weight easier and quicker.

Don't worry, we'll get into easy exercises and simple diet changes later in the book. For now, just take note of these tips and think about which ones you can start using in your daily life today.

36

AROUND THE HOUSE

There are always things that need to be done around the house, aren't there?

Well gues what? Doing basic chores and things around the house can help you lose weight too. It keeps you moving, keeps you motivated, and keeps you thinking "what next?".

I always feel great after cleaning the house and organizing things. I start to do some simple sweeping, then I get out the vacuum. After that, I begin to organize and reorganize my rooms, office, living area. Larger items and chairs and desks and furniture gets moved. It's like a fun workout!

Another thing I've done is I keep more plants around the house. They look great, and some plants smell great - and I'm able to take a walk around the house watering the plants. Although it's not crunches or treadmill running, these little things can keep you going throughout the day without feeling overwhelmed.

Find some things you can do around the house that aren't too overwhelming but will help you lose weight and help the house stay clean and organized.

37

STAIRS INSTEAD OF ELEVATOR

This is a tip that you've heard time and time again, and I'm including it because of how important it is for both your physical body and mental state of mind.

Taking the stairs instead of the elevator is something we all want to do, but most of us don't. Reason being - It's so easy to choose the easy way out; I mean come on, the elevator was invented for the reason of not having to take the stairs!

Losing weight isn't easy. It's simple, but it isn't easy. When you have the choice of stairs or elevator, make the conscious choice of taking the stairs.

First of all, you will be working out, moving your legs, working your muscles all around your body, as well as getting a nice short swift cardio workout. And second, choosing the slightly more difficult route will again program your mind to think of obstacles in a different way. You have the willpower to choose stairs over elevator, and next will be choosing a healthier meal, and after that will be choosing a harder workout, and soon it will be choosing to be thin.

Losing the weight starts with the choices you make. Whether big or small, start making the choices that are truly going to benefit you and your life.

38

PARKING FURTHER AWAY

Like choosing the stairs instead of the elevator, this involves giving yourself an easy, swift workout and cardio while doing a normal daily task.

Have you ever seen a handicapped person pull into a handicapped spot in front, only to find out that they are only handicapped because they chose to overeat and not take care of themselves? If you've been to a comedy club before, you've probably heard the joke about how 'fat people should have to park at the back so they can get a workout'. Funnyness or rudeness aside, it's true.

If all overweight people parked in the final last spots, furthest away from the store they were going to; little by little, they would lose weight. Instead of the average weight being 150 pounds, maybe it would be 145 pounds. Again, I'm not saying that you will shave off any number of pounds by parking furthest away a certain amount of times. However, it's one of those things that works out your body because of the brief walk, and works out your mind because of you choosing to make a decision that will benefit your future self more than your present self.

39

PLAY WITH KIDS MORE

Play with the kids more. And if you don't have kids, then just play (physical activity, not video games) in general. Maybe you have a brother or sister or friend you can play with.

Do you know why some kids get fat while others stay skinny? It has a lot to do with the parents sadly. Children don't just become fat. They play less, then don't play at all. They eat more than others, then eat other's food, then eat much more than others. They have snacks when others don't. They don't get active with friends.

Overweight kids don't need a professional workout routine and diet plan, they need to play more and just get active. And that is something that we as adults can use ourselves. How fun would it be to swing on a tire swing, or slide down a slide? How about playing catch with a football, or a frisbee?

There are hundreds of things you can do and play that keeps you active, keeps you having fun, and helps you lose weight while not having to even think about it.

40

BECOME A DIY PERSON

Got projects?

If you aren't a DIY person, become one. If you are a DIY person, do more projects!

DIY stands for do-it-yourself, and what I'm getting at is you doing some projects around the house, get yourself sweating a little bit.

You can build a birdhouse. You can fix your door knob or your creaky hinges. You could get into welding or soldering and metalwork your way to some cool art. Build a planterbox or do some other type of woodworking.

The possibilities are endless with DIY projects, and they are great because you can do advanced projects or be a complete beginner and still do enough work to break a sweat, feel accomplished, get something done, and lose a little weight in the process.

And take note: You don't have to do any huge daunting projects if you don't want to. It can be as simple as painting or knitting. I would recommend doing something that allows you to stand, move around, move your arms and legs, but just doing something is important enough.

41

WASH YOUR CAR

How's your car looking? Maybe you haven't washed it in awhile.

Maybe your car is looking great, but only because the guys down at the car wash did a great job last week.

Instead of not washing your car or letting someone else wash your car, you wash the car. If you've never washed your own car before, it's easy and doesn't have to be complicated at all. Start with a running water hose, a bucket, sponge, and soap (basic soap is fine, you can upgrade to the auto stuff later). If you want to clean the inside, get a vacuum out as well.

Washing your car inside and out is a nice little exercise that you can do weekly or even every 2 weeks. And if you have multiple cars or family's cars, you can wash those as well and spend some more time exercising.

Just like any other physical activity, this gets your heart rate going, can get you sweating, moves your muscles around to avoid stiffness or restlessness, and of course can help you lose weight.

42

AVOID SITTING AROUND

I wanted to save this tip for the last of this "daily routine" section of the book. This might sound self explanatory, but it finishes off this section nicely by summing up why it's important you don't sit around for long periods of time.

The more you are just sitting there, the easier it is to not get up, and the harder it feels to get up. It's like the typical "get out of bed in the morning" syndrome. You wake up, and immediately you feel the warmth underneath the covers. The longer you lay under the covers, the colder it feels every time you are about to take them off to get out of bed.

If you don't need to sit, then don't sit. If you can go most of the day standing or walking around, do it. Of course there will always be those relaxing times of the day where you just want to sit back and relax for a little while - but don't turn your relaxing time into a wasted day.

WEIGHT LOSS, DIET AND FOOD

You have a plan, and you have the motivation and mindset. You also have some nice daily routine tips to follow.

Now comes the meat to the book with our final two sections: Diet & Food and Exercise & Fitness.

This is section 4, Diet and Food, and is the largest section of the book. Although there are tons of things we can do and change to lose weight, the one thing that will always remain as the culprit of gaining weight is FOOD.

If you can control the type of food and amount of it that goes into your system, and you also know how you are using that food to produce energy, you will be able to lose weight much easier. When you can control your diet, everything else on top of it will just quicken the weight loss process.

Some of these tips are short and sweet, while others have a bit more detail to them - but all of them are important. Follow along with the tips, take some notes, and start taking these diet and food tips into consideration.

43

CHEW THOROUGHLY

Did your parents or grandparents ever tell you to chew your food 50 or 100 or more times before you swallowed?

Sometimes their reason is it enhances the flavor, some said it allows you to enjoy every bite of your food, others say it has to do with pacing your eating and letting your brain catch up with your stomach.

Whatever the reason, chewing your food thoroughly can do all of these things, and generally puts more time into eating while eating the same amount. When you pace yourself like this, your brain really does have more time to then realize that your stomach is full and you probably shouldn't have seconds or eat further.

So next time you are at the dinner table, make each bite count, and try to pace yourself enough so that you feel full and satisfied without overeating.

44

A NOTE ABOUT OATS

Why are oats so good for losing weight?

Well, you may or may not know that they are rich in fiber, which can make you feel more full than you really are.

Although oats have more carbohydrates than other food, it also burns fat and boosts your metabolism because they are what we call a "slow digesting food".

Besides having a lot of fiber, they won't have too much of an impact on your blood sugar either. Most oats are very healthy for you, but watch out for the PROCESSED oats. Say NO to that instant oatmeal crud, and get some real oats or oat groats (crushed grainy oats).

45

FAT FREE ISN'T SUGAR FREE

"Oh look, fat free! Perfect!"

Think again... Fat free doesn't mean sugar free, and sugar can be an overweight person's worst enemy.

Although sugar doesn't contain fat itself, it can contribute to the creation of fat (yes, your body will actually turn sugar into fat).

Glucose, even though it is a simple sugar and important energy source, it also has it's detriments. Pack your body with sugar, and you'll have more energy/fuel than you need. So what happens to the excess? Your liver converts the sugar into fatty acids and pumps it right back into your bloodstream. Your blood stream will then pump these fatty acids all over your body, giving you a nasty new layer of fat.

So keep in mind that fat free doesn't mean you can't gain fat weight from it. Although it doesn't start as fat, it will end as fat.

46

PORTION SIZE CONTROL

Do you realize how messed up our portions have gotten over the years?

Back in the day we used to have a small hamburger or sandwich with a small handful of fries and a pint or smaller sized cup of juice or soda. Today we have large burgers, huge sandwiches, almost full plates of greasy fries.

Even eating out has gotten a little out of control. At almost every place I've been to in the past 5 years, I can split up my meal into 3 or 4 separate meals and have a separate dinner for half the week or more.

Overweight people ask me why I don't finish my meals, and act as if it is a crime if anything is left over. Then I look at their belly, and bite my tongue thinking they probably aren't the best candidates for talking about how much someone should or shouldn't eat.

You don't have to finish your entire plate, we're not in the Great Depression anymore. In fact, when you get your dinner, ask for a to-go box upfront. Put half or more of your meal into this box, and you'll be surprised to find out that you feel more than full after finishing your "full meal", while you hadn't really even finished half of it yet.

There's nothing better than losing weight AND saving money at the same time (all while savoring a delicious meal more than once).

47

GROCERY LISTS N' LIMITS

It's grocery shopping time again, and you're getting ready to get in the car to head to the store.

But wait! First you need to set up a list and some limits.

Earlier we talked about how you shouldn't go grocery shopping on an empty stomach, as it could entice you to buy fatty foods that will fill you up instead of the healthier (and still filling) choices around you.

Besides that, you must have a grocery list if you want to stick to the healthier choices. Without one, it is easier to fall into the trap of buying what looks good rather than what you really need.

Once you make your grocery list, you should also set up a time limit for your grocery run. 30 minutes is usually enough time to shop for at least a few days to a week or more. If you need more time, that's fine, just set up a limit. The reason you should set up a time limit is because even with a list; once the list is completed, you are then free to roam the store and scrounge for "whatever else you want". Don't do this!

Setting up a time limit allows you to get in, get what you need, and get out. You'll feel great, you won't waste a lot of time, you'll save money, and you will surely be helping yourself lose weight in the process.

48

APPLES AND BANANAS

I like to eat, eat, eat, apples and bananas!

You've probably heard the song before. But even for how catchy the song is, so many of us don't eat enough fresh fruits, especially apples and bananas.

Yes, apples and bananas have carbs, which can be our worst enemy. However, there IS such a thing as good carbs.

Everything is either fat, protein, or carbs, or a combo. Sure fruit has carbs, it also has SUGAR! However, apples and bananas also have fiber, and can make you again feel more full than you already are.

Forget about large processed breakfast cereals and other morning food. Instead, eat 1 apple or 1 banana and you'll be suprised at how long you can go without really feeling hungry again.

49

WATER BEFORE BREAKFAST

Water is the best thing for you. It's also the one thing we absolutely need in order to survive.

Having a glass of water in the morning makes your skin glow, renews cells in your body, can help cure illnesses, balances the lymph system, purifies the colon, and yes you guessed it - can also help you LOSE WEIGHT!

When you have water right when you wake up in the morning (1 glass is fine, 2 glasses or about 16 ounces is better), you will boost your body's metabolism (by as much as 25% or more), helping you crush the fat that enters and forms in your body.

Better yet, add a squeeze of lemon in your water, and you'll cleanse your system, help your body digest food easier, boost your immune system, lose weight (fiber fiber fiber!), and give you a boost of energy. Adding lemon also gives you that boost without the need for caffeine (say NO to coffee!), giving you energy without the crash later.

50

WATER-RICH FOODS

Most water rich foods are fruits and vegetables, which can be great for losing weight (and the general health of your body).

Water-rich foods contain fiber, vitamins, and antioxidants, and keeps your body hydrated just like water does. Many detox and cleansing diets promote water-rich foods as well.

So... what types of foods are rich in water? The best are fruits and veggies. Here's some examples:

Fruits: watermelon, strawberries, grapefruit, apricots, pineapple, cantaloupe, oranges.

Veggies: Tomato, celery, cucumber, broccoli, eggplant, radishes, zucchini.

When you think about it, and really when you actually taste these fruits and veggies, you can really tell that they are full of water.

So, when you are thinking of having some fruits and veggies, try choosing from this list first.

51

EAT AT HOME

Earlier we talked about how you can use portion control to your advantage at restaurants.

Well what's even better than controlling your portions at restaurants is controlling your portions at home. Eating at home allows you to cook a specific amount of something and know exactly what you are cooking.

If you don't know how to cook, it might be time to learn (it can be a great hobby, and can help you learn about a variety of healthy but delicious cooking choices).

Let's say you cook a pasta that can be broken up into anywhere between 4 to 10 servings. Choose how much you want to eat tonight, and then put away the rest into separate containers. Buy lots of containers so you can have lots of different measured portions of food that you can heat up any time you want.

You can always have a pre-portioned healthy delicious snack or meal whenever you want by stacking many different portioned meals into your fridge. Just make sure you eat them before they go bad, stale or rotten.

52

MORE SNACKS! (WHAT?)

Want to lose more weight? Eat more snacks!

Seriously, eating more snacks can help you lose weight. But how?

It's not that eating more will help you lose more weight. This involves eating more frequently during the day but in smaller portions.

When you eat those large dinners (or even breakfasts or lunches), you are stretching your stomach. You overfill yourself with food, only to later feel even more hungry because your stomach is a little larger than it was a few hours ago.

By skipping out on the large meals and portion controlling your day into smaller snacks, you can keep your stomach from stretching out, causing you to WANT to eat less, which helps immensely when you are trying to shave off the weight.

Think about how this can effect your future as time goes on. By eating smaller snacks, you can decrease your food consumption by at least 25% for sure. This will stretch your stomach 25% less of the time, giving your mind more times to say "I don't need food right now, my stomach is quite full".

53

ADD SOME PEPPER

Not from the pepper shaker, ACTUAL peppers. Yes, the hot ones.

Peppers contain "capsaicin", which is what gives peppers that HOT flavor.

Without going into scientific detail, our bodies contain both white fat cells and brown fat cells. Too much white fat causes us to become obese (or at least put on those extra pounds).

Brown fat is highly active and "regulates body temperature". Studies have shown that after direct exposure to capsaicin (hot peppers), brown fat activity was higher.

So what does this brown fat do? Well, although it won't burn off the fat 10 pounds at a time with doing nothing else, it can increase the amount of calories you burn during normal daily activity. Combine that with some cardio and exercise, and you have a nice match.

54

FRESH FRUIT > FRUIT JUICE

Have you looked at all the ADDITIVES they put into fruit juice these days?

It's really sad when you pick up a container that clearly says "FRUIT JUICE" on it, but then in tiny writing at the bottom or back it says "less than 1% juice".

So what is the rest of the 99% of the crap inside the juice container? Well, it's different for all juices, but most of the time it doesn't provide any further or greater benefit than by eating the actual fruit itself.

This also goes for eating fresh fruit rather than eating yogurt with "fruit added". You can buy some low fat plain yogurt and add your own fresh fruit to it and have a delicious yet very healthy snack.

Avoid the sugar, avoid the syrup, avoid the dye, avoid the additives. Just stick with fresh fruit. Although don't think that fresh fruit has no consequences either. You can overdo anything, and eating fruit is included. Eat too much and you will gain weight, but eat the same amount of fresh fruit as you would fruit juice, and you'll lose weight (or it will at least help).

55

CUT DOWN ON ALCOHOL

If you are currently overweight (you must be if you are reading this book), then you should really just cut out alcohol all together.

Yeah yeah, you hear about the "beer belly". But what does that even mean?

Calories are just the "energy" that exist in edible food/liquid. More calories consumed means more energy into your body. Alcohol has a TON of calories.

But really what happens (or doesn't happen) is while your body processes the alcohol, it stops processing fat. And by processing, I don't mean it doesn't consume any fat, I mean it doesn't BURN any fat. It is only once the ethanol from the alcohol is completely gone and out of your system when you are able to start burning fat again.

So if you are one of those heavy partiers who drinks every night, and then also the next day, you could be setting your entire body up for failure, because you will hardly ever be able to burn any fat or calories in order to lose weight at all. So why do the Jersey Shore guys (the show, not the place) get to drink all day and night and they have ripped bodies and six pack abs? Because they also work out and exercise heavily, and probably work on a whole lot of other stuff to keep their bodies looking the way they want.

You may have heard of studies that say that alcohol can make you LOSE weight! But, with every theory and study, there has never been a solid answer. Drinking alcohol can actually make you more hungry, not to mention the time lost in your weight loss journey. Drink some alcohol and then go run a mile (yeah right...).

Beer has a Glycaemic Index of 119, while wine and spirits have a GI of 0. I'm not saying to go drink a whole bottle of wine tonight (for the other facts about alcohol in general), but beer is probably the worst for you out of any alcohol.

Amy Culderson and Mike Shaw

Just cut down (or cut out) on the alcohol from your life, and you will see faster results with your weight loss progress, and it will be easier to burn fat and calories.

56

AVOIDING MAYONNAISE

Mayo has lots of fat and lots of calories, avoid it at all costs.

Americans love mayonnaise. Why do you think most of us are overweight? Okay, so it's not because of mayo entirely, but it does have it's big disadvantages to losing weight.

Most mayonnaise distributors produce mayonnaise with high saturated fat content. Add that on top of what you usually put mayonnaise on (white bread and some sort of meat for a sandwich or burger), and you have a whopping fat meal.

Look, mayonnaise isn't going to make or break you, but cutting it out will help you lose weight faster and easier.

You can eat 10 sandwiches packed with mayo in one day - and as long as you are able to burn off all of those calories, you won't gain any weight. Take this tip into consideration. Some will say "mayo doesn't make ME gain weight, in fact when I STOPPED eating mayo I STARTED gaining weight!" - Well, maybe because they traded the mayo for worse things. But if you just get rid of mayo and don't add any other calories into your meal, it will help.

57

NO MORE COFFEE

It's actually quite funny to hear all of the conflicting arguments made for not just coffee but many other weight loss tips and fads.

Right now I'm reading an article of a man who claims drinking coffee 4 times a day made him lose weight. Let's laugh out loud together - lol.

Look, coffee CAN give you a boost of caffeine which, yes, can get you moving faster. But what about the calories in coffee? What about the crash later that makes you feel tired and lazy? Trust me, take my tip from earlier and drink LEMON WATER instead of coffee, and you'll feel much better (as it is infinitely better for you).

Coffee makes our body produce cortisol, which many call the "stress hormone". Cortisol increases your blood sugar, which is then turned into fat.

Drink coffee long enough (every day for years), and your body will begin to relocate this newly created fat into your abdomen, which will begin to give you a beer belly, or what you can now call a coffee belly.

Just get rid of coffee already, as well as anything else with heightened levels of caffeine.

Now... if you are falling asleep during the day and your job or life depends on you pumping some caffeine into your system to stay awake so you won't lose your job or worse fall asleep while driving or operating machinery, then by all means drink the damn coffee. Many only come up with excuses as to why they can't do it. I'm here to tell you that you can.

58

EVER TRY SKIMMED MILK?

The argument now continues in this book regarding skimmed milk VS fat free milk.

Skim milk is not fat free milk, as some would suggest - it's actually better in a way. Both skim milk and fat free milk will be better than whole milk if we are talking about losing weight.

It's easy to put it this way: Whole milk contains MORE fat, but also MORE dairy nutrients. Fat-free milk contains NO fat and much less nutrients. SKIMMED milk contains lower than half a percent of milk fat, which is more than 0 fat, BUT it also gives you the nutrients you want and need without packing on the extra calories, fat and cholesterol.

So, skim milk can actually be your best bet, because you are still getting the nutrients and calcium that your body needs while cutting down on the fat that whole milk contains.

59

AVOID PROCESSED FOODS

I'm not even just talking about "junk food" here. You might not even know about some highly processed foods.

We know why processed foods and ingredients are bad - I mean come on, it's in the word - they are PROCESSED, meaning they were created by humans in a lab (as opposed to getting natural ingredients that already exist in the world).

You might not be able to cut out ALL processed foods, but you will lose weight if you cut down on them.

Here's some processed foods to look out for (that you might not have even known about):

Artificial ingredients (red 40, blue 1, artificial sweeteners). Refined sweeteners are also bad (try natural honey instead!). Dump the 'refined grains' and go for whole-grain.

Factory farmed animals have completely unnatural diets and are given synthetic hormones to produce meat quickly and efficiently (instead of healthily and for-the-people). Forget canola oil and go for butter or olive oil.

Stay away from pre-flavored packaged products (get it plain and add your own natural flavor to it). Low-fat and fat-free products seem like a win, but since they take away the tasty fat, they now have to pack it with sugar, which as you've learned the excess sugar gets turned into fat anyway (and in many cases equals out to MORE fat than the regular 'fat' food).

And I don't even need to tell you about fast food... Jeeze Laweeze, Americans... the proof is right in front of us. Fast food = Fast fat.

The more natural and healthy you can get your food, the better it is for you, and the faster you'll lose weight (and in a completely natural and healthy way).

60

REMOVE SKIN FROM CHICKEN

This is just a quick tip, but do you know how much fat is in just the SKIN of chicken?

Answer: Not any more than the rest of the chicken - that is... UNTIL IT IS COOKED!

As soon as you start to cook chicken with the skin ON, the skin will act like a fat magnet, pulling up and sucking in ALL of those fatty oils right into the skin.

Well, that doesn't happen as much with chicken with the skin OFF. Take the skin off your chicken, cook it, eat it. This is just another little thing you can do to help lose the weight faster.

61

HYDRATE ALL DAY LONG

You know that water first thing in the morning (with a zing of lemon of course!) is good for you, but it's also important to hydrate yourself all day long.

Studies have shown that those who drink water right before their meals lost around 29% more weight (over the course of a few months).

Firstly, drinking more water right before meals makes you less hungry, allowing you to stop yourself before you start to overeat.

On top of that, drinking water before during and after meals helps you digest your food easier. This helps you not just lose weight but also keeps you more energized and awake throughout the day.

Here's some more quick tips on how you can use water to your advantage: Replace sweet drinks with water, and drink cold water (studies show it speeds up metabolism). For any alcohol you drink (if you must drink alcohol), match it with an equal amount of water to get the alcohol in and out as soon as possible. Finally, cut down on the salt/sodium as much as you can as you increase your water intake, and it will help you lose "water weight" quicker.

62

EAT MORE PROTEIN

Okay okay, before you go tell all your friends that you're going to eat giant bowls of mozzarella cheese all day to lose weight, hear me out...

The title says "eat more protein", but what that means is you need to cut down on sweets, fried foods, and grain based foods.

Essentially, protein helps build and maintain muscle while helping to lose fat.

So put it this way: You can eat the same amount of sugary sweets and the same amount of protein to keep the results you are getting (losing or barely maintaining muscle while gaining fat). But in order to drop the FAT while maintaining the muscle, you can in fact DOUBLE your protein intake while cutting in HALF your intake of processed foods, sugary sweets, and other fat-gaining foods and drinks.

Don't go overboard though, and remember that just because something has protein in it does not necessarily mean that it doesn't have fat or sugar or carbs in it as well.

63

AVOID TOO MUCH SALT/SODIUM

Yes, salt and sodium is NEEDED in order to live.

Salt retains water and allows your body to function. Electrolytes (salt has em') trigger us to consume more water, prevents your muscles from cramping, keeps good minerals in your bloodstream, and contains vital nutrients that help maintain your digestive system. A lack of salt is dangerous, no doubt.

However, TOO MUCH of it can pack on the pounds.

Salt triggers your body to release dopamine (the pleasure neurotransmitter) which makes you crave even more salt (similar to alcohol and nicotine). This would be okay but... think about the different types of salty foods that exist - pretzels, potato chips, processed food, fast food. You'll crave it more, you'll eat it more, and you'll gain more weight.

You already know that salt increases thirst (that's why bars and pubs give away nuts and chips and pretzels and ANYTHING with salt for free, so you DRINK more). It would be nice to think that when we are thirsty we'd drink water only, but you know that's not the case. Most turn to sugary drinks, soda, juice (with no real juice in it), alcohol - you get the picture, all the stuff that makes you gain fat.

One salt tip you might not know is that it produces insulin, which basically tells your body to store any excess/additional sugar as fat (remember when you learned about sugar turning into fat?).

So yes, you need SOME salt in order to live. But if you are like most people, I'm sure you are already getting an excess of salt, so CUT IT DOWN! More salt means more hunger, more thirst, more sugar, more fat, and more weight.

64

MORE WHOLE GRAINS

Once again, these are one of those things that are good for you, but have too much and it could go the other way fast.

What type of bread do you eat? Many choose white bread (made with white flour). Switching out all of your white bread with whole grain bread is a healthy choice.

However, just because it is better doesn't mean it is the best. Some whole grain food is also packed with sugar and sodium (and you just learned about sodium!).

Forget chips and crackers, no matter how "whole grain" they are - Those companies still need to make their money, so they'll pack in whatever they can to make their "healthy whole grain snack" salty, sugary and deliciously fat.

Go for brown rice instead of white rice, whole-grain/whole-wheat bread instead of white bread, and oatmeal instead of sugary cereal.

Whole grains allow your body to feel more full, which allows you to feel less hungry throughout the day. They are naturally low in fat, with no cholesterol, contain good protein, and gives you lots of fiber.

65

LESS SODA (NONE!)

Here's a VERY quick tip. Don't drink soda!!

I don't care if it says "diet". I don't care if it says "0 calories". I don't care if it says "caffeine free".

Even with a "Diet Caffeine Free 0 Calorie No Fat" soda, you are still hurting your chances at losing weight by drinking this stuff.

That diet caffeine free no calorie soda still contains: carbonation, aspartame, sodium, acid, phenylalanine, and other "crap". Too much soda can lead to diabetes, can make you fat, destroy your teeth, increase your blood pressure, increases risk for kidney stones, and most of the time contains high fructose corn syrup or artificial sweetener.

No where on any soda does it say "healthy". I've never seen a soda that helps you lose weight (even though they 'tried' by throwing the word DIET on the bottle). On most soda bottles I see, they almost all say "NOT a significant source of fat calories, saturated fat, trans fat, cholesterol, fiber, sugars, vitamin A, vitamin C, calcium and iron".

Besides wanting to lose weight, you should also want to be healthy while you do it, and drinking soda is a HUGE no-no if you are going for health and natural ingredients.

Just stop drinking soda, it's actually not that hard. Get 100% juice, or better yet, WATER!

66

COOK WITH NO OIL

If you can cook with no oil at all, do it.

Okay okay, so you might not be able to cook with 'no' oil, but you CAN cook with healthy oils!

When I mean healthy, I mean high in healthy fat and low in saturated fat.

Some safe and healthy cooking oils include: Macadamia Nut Oil, Peanut Oil, Olive Oil, Avocado Oil, and if we count fats you can use butter, ghee and lard as well (don't worry, just because it's 'fat' doesn't mean it's not healthy fat).

But my favorite-tasting AND safest AND most fat-burning oil out there is... COCONUT OIL! This is one of the healthiest oils for you, and can lower cholesterol, boost your activeness energy and alertness, helps prevent disease, and is also the safest due to it's VERY high cooking temperature allowance.

Now if you want to use an oil besides these, just make sure it is NOT any of the following: Canola oil, soybean oil, corn oil, or sunflower oil.

67

CHOOSING PROTEIN SOURCES

As you previously learned, increased protein while cutting back on sugars fats and carbs can help you lose weight. It also promotes good health in your system.

However, not all protein sources are created equally.

When choosing protein sources, go for carbs that are high in fiber (whole grains, fruits and veggies). I also recommend chicken (with no skin of course), LEAN beef (not too much though), low-fat dairy, pork, and fish.

Don't go overboard on protein though, or you might not get enough vitamins and minerals that other foods offer. However, you can always take a multivitamin to balance that.

A lot of what dieting comes down to is finding a healthy balance. Take in the good protein, but don't make it the only thing you consume. Find a healthy medium that works for you.

68

LESS SUGARY BEVERAGES

I'm not even talking about soda anymore, we both know soda is bad.

But what's funny is... Some FRUIT drinks are even worse!

I'm looking at this "fruit energy drink" that has 56 grams of sugar! You know that "Arizona Half and Half Lemonade/Iced Tea? 39 grams of sugar. This Sobe Citrus drink has 76 grams of sugar. Do I need go on?

I've told you a few times now - Excess sugar doesn't just flow through and out of your system. It turns into fat! There's also dozens of other health risks that come with high-sugar drinks.

Next time you pick up any beverage, take a look at the sugar content. If it doesn't state it, don't think that means it's a 0... haha. Look it up on the internet, and you'll be morbidly disgusted.

If you are going to go for a sugary beverage at all, go for 100% fruit juice with REAL sugar instead of the processed crap that's all over the place these days. Yes, they will be hard to find, but once you find one or two, you'll notice them every time you go to the store.

SIDE FACT: I'm laughing right now because earlier today I witnessed a 400 pound (give or take 50 pounds) man fill up the "X-TREME Big Gulp" at 7-11 with Coca Cola. Guess how much sugar is in this drink that this guy was probably going to finish by the end of his meal? 150 damn grams of sugar. Come on people, just stop.

69

EATING RAW FOODS

I'm not going to go too much into depth with this, or even promote a 100% raw foods diet.

Some have had success with completely raw foods, but most I know have not.

Basically, the 100% raw foodists believe that heating up food completely kills the natural enzymes and nutrients they once contained. These enzymes and nutrients can help boost your immune system, get rid of allergies and headaches, improve your health, and in our case, LOSE WEIGHT.

However, if you go 100% raw, you are leaving out the much needed protein, vitamins, calcium, B12, iron, and other minerals your body needs. Sure you can take supplements and vitamins and even protein powder (and other powder or pills or meal replacements), but it's easier to just do both.

You can have the best of both worlds, no one is stopping you. Cook your chicken for protein, get your fish and lean meat and other foods you cook. Then, you can also add on the raw foods - unprocessed, organic (for the most part), non-cooked. All fruits and veggies are raw foods. Grains, nuts and seeds. Even raw fish and raw eggs are considered part of the raw foods diet.

If you can stick to more raw foods and less processed foods, it is almost a guarantee that you will lose weight quicker (and still be healthy and safe while doing it). However, the more raw you get and the less you cook, the more of a necessity it is to learn about what essentials you'll be missing out on.

Find your own happy medium between raw foods and cooked foods, but at all costs do what you can do avoid processed foods.

70

A NOTE ABOUT SALADS

It's hard for people to stick with the super basic salad, but it's also detrimental to your weight loss journey to have a large salad with lots of calories, added ingredients, fattening dressings, salt and pepper, and more.

So what's my "note about salads"? Well, it's a few notes actually.

First of all, the tips I'm about to give you also depend on whether you are making the salad yourself or ordering it from a restaurant.

If you are preparing the salad yourself, you will be able to follow all of these tips easily. If you are ordering from a restaurant, it requires a little more willpower.

Let's talk about the TYPE of lettuce/greens in your salad. If you are making it yourself, I suggest mixing lots of different greens into one salad, including basil and/or parsley and other herbs. You'll get more nutrients and antioxidants (as well as some nice natural flavors). If you are ordering out, just get the 'garden salad' or 'mixed greens'.

You can add cheese, but not too much. Cheese is calcium, and calcium releases fat. But add too much cheese, and you'll pack on extra calories that you don't need. Cheese is good, just go light on it.

Adding chicken or salmon is a nice way to pump up the protein, but like I stated before, these foods have other ingredients besides the main one (being protein in this case). Keep it small, but feel free to add some chicken or fish into your salad. And if you're really ready to add some more goodness to your salad, chop up some fruits and/or veggies into your salad as well.

Finally, try using an oil-based salad dressing (and even some vinegar) and ditch the creamy opaque dressings (as opposed to more transparent). However, you DO NOT need to go fat-free with this, in fact I recommend you don't! Your body won't be able to absorb the other vitamins and nutrients that are in your salad without at least some fat in there. Not only does this increase the nutrients and vitamins your body absorbs, but it also fills you up faster, allowing you to not overeat.

One more tip: NO CROUTONS!!! They seem harmless enough, but croutons (especially the white-bread ones) have hardly any nutrients or anything useful to your body, and can actually increase your blood sugar (which can lead to excess sugar being turned into fat, not to mention many other health risks).

71

FOCUS ON YOUR MEAL

This short tip is called "focusing on your meal".

Do you find that while you are eating, whether it's breakfast lunch or dinner, that you don't even think about eating, you just... eat?

We've eaten food so regularly in our lives that we don't even think about when we eat, what we eat, how we eat, or how much we eat. We just eat when we THINK we are hungry.

Like chewing your food thoroughly, focus on your entire meal, think about how much is in front of you. Put your fork down between bites, or if it's finger food - put your burger or sandwich down after every bite, don't keep it sitting in your hand. When a fork or piece of food stays in your hand, you are telling yourself to continue, continue, continue eating.

Envision all the food on your plate fitting in your stomach. Do you really want to stuff that much into your body? How much weight do you want to gain tonight? Focus on your meal, and understand that it's okay to tell the rest of your meal "no, I'll eat you another time".

72

2 Minute Meal Break

I love this rule, I call it the 2 minute meal break.

This goes with focusing on your meal and other 'during the meal' tips, and it involves taking a quick 2 minute break where you don't eat anything during your meal to evaluate a few things.

You are evaluating... How much you have eaten, if you are still hungry right now, if you can fit anymore into your stomach, how long of an exercise or workout you must do later in order to burn these calories.

When you take a quick break in the middle of your meal, you are again "allowing your mind to catch up with your stomach". More times than not, when I take a meal break, I find out that I'm stuffed and save the rest of my delicious food for a second (and sometimes 3rd) meal the next day.

73

NEVER STARVE YOURSELF

I know I've talked a lot about how eating less will help you lose weight. Of course it will, but that doesn't mean you should ever starve yourself.

This is probably self-explanatory to most, but it's worth talking about. Many previously overweight people fall into the trap of eating disorders, and end up starving themselves for days just so they can lose a few pounds.

Starving yourself or not eating food when you are actually hungry can hurt you more than it can help you. There have been full length books written on this very subject, so I won't have time to go over everything that "could" happen. But what I can tell you is, it's important to have the happy medium. Work out, exercise, eat healthy, move around during the day, change your thoughts, feelings, actions, your routine.

You can lose all the weight you want, and you'll never have to starve yourself, ever. Remember that.

74

EAT MORE TIMES IN A DAY

That's right, instead of starving yourself, EAT MORE times during the day.

You learned about eating smaller meals or snacking during the day (healthy snacks of course), now let's talk about eating more frequently during the day in general.

This is what most people call grazing, taken from how cows and/or goats graze and chew/eat grass all day long. Of course you don't want to weigh as much as a cow, but the grazing still works for us humans.

Each time you eat, your stomach expands. When the energy and 'stuff' from the food is broken down inside and given to your body (and some that comes out of your body), your stomach takes longer to detract to it's original state.

So if you eat 4 large meals during the day, you are constantly stretching and expanding your stomach, giving you the urge to eat more because your mind believes your stomach is more empty and needs food.

But if you break those meals into two, and eat 8 smaller meals during the day, your stomach doesn't stretch as much, making you feel less hungry during the day. You might not even get to your 7th or 8th meal because you feel fine (and still energized enough to workout and do your normal daily routine).

75

EAT AT THE SAME TIMES

Does your schedule fluctuate? That's okay, you can still make time to eat (just like we HAVE to make time to sleep).

Remember when you learned it's a bad idea to work in the kitchen/dining room, and a bad idea to eat in your office or where you work? Same idea with eating at the same times during the day.

When you have somewhat of a set schedule for when you eat during the day, you don't feel hungry during the rest of the time during your day.

Now, you don't have to punch your time card for your 5 minute snack in the afternoon (you don't have to plan your really small snacks). But try scheduling 30 minutes or an hour for lunch, then a specific hour or two time slot for dinner.

After a few days pass, then a few weeks, your mind and body will know your schedule and habitual actions, and during the daily times where you hadn't eaten anything previously during that time for weeks, your mind will tell yourself that you are not hungry, because it is not time to eat.

76

Conscious Calorie Intake

Calories, calories, calories. It seems like everyone's talking about calories.

Well, it's because if you can control the intake of calories into your system, you can control much more precisely your weight fluctuations and changes.

Next time you pick up any piece of food (or even drink, don't forget beverages have calories too!), take a look at how many calories it has.

You can use a calorie calculator that bases your recommended calorie intake on your age, gender, weight, height, and exercise level (and much more on more advanced sites and apps). However, if you want a general idea, it is recommended for men to have about 2,500 calories per day and women 2,000 calories per day.

You need calories to survive. Don't think you can cut your calories close to 0 and expect to lose weight. You'll soon pass out within a few days, and could not just pass out, but pass away for good.

However, use the 2,500 for men and 2,000 for women daily calorie estimates, and do your best to NOT go over your daily recommended amount.

Try limiting or avoiding the following foods in order to limit your calorie intake: animal fats, lard, vegetable oils, salad dressing, snacks, candies, cheese, processed meats, fried foods.

The more you can avoid or limit the intake of these types of foods, the easier it will be for you to lose weight.

SCARY FACT/TIP: Stay away from fast food alltogether. Did you know, if you are a woman who has a daily recommended calorie intake of 1,800 calories, it's easy to pass up that calorie level with just 1 fast food meal? Crazy, but completely true and something you should think about.

77

GREEN TEA WEIGHT LOSS

Green tea is awesome, and I'll drink it over coffee any day of the week.

Green tea fights heart disease and cancer, and will also help fight fat as well.

"Catechins" are found in green tea, which stimulate your body to burn more calories (which essentially decreases body fat).

Don't settle for other "teas" either. Black tea and Oolong tea come from the same "Camellia Sinensis" plant that green tea does. However, green tea leaves are NOT fermented before steaming and drying (unlike the others), which helps your body burn fat and lower cholesterol.

78

TRY A HEAVY BREAKFAST

It's called the "Big Breakfast Diet", and basically it calls for eating a larger breakfast, but then a smaller lunch and dinner.

Usually, most of us can't do this for the fact that we live with at least one other person who probably isn't on the same diet as us. So you can't expect to eat a large breakfast alone, and then watch your family and/or friends wine and dine in front of you for dinner while you eat hardly anything.

However, if you know you are able to eat big early and eat small later, then I say go for it. This doesn't mean eating unhealthy though, as some who follow the big breakfast diet claim.

For breakfast, you are to have protein, carbohydrates and fats, and sweets. Then for lunch and dinner, you CANNOT have ANY carbs or sweets.

What this big breakfast diet helps you do is boost your metabolism early on so that you don't have the craving for sweets and other treats later in the day.

79

GOOD MULTIVITAMIN SUPPLEMENT

I don't need to go over this too much, as you should definitely be taking some sort of daily vitamin each day.

Vitamins give you the nutrients that most of us don't receive through the food we eat (or don't eat) during the day. All vitamins are different, but a simple "one-a-day" type multi-vitamin supplement is a good start.

Take your vitamin(s) in the morning. When you take it, you are giving yourself energy, vitamins, nutrients. You are packing your body with the good stuff, and again you are telling your mind "I now have these nutrients, therefore I don't feel hungry because I don't need anything extra". I don't recommend a vitamin without food or water, but you'll find that taking a vitamin daily can keep you more energized during the day and in the big picture help you lose weight.

80

HIGH IN FIBER

We've gone over certain fruits, veggies, and other food that contains fiber, but why is fiber so good for you, especially when trying to lose weight?

Fiber actually does not break down and absorb into your body at all. In fact, it passes fast right through your digestive tract, without breaking down much at all.

YES, THIS is why when we eat a lot of fiber, we have more of a need to go to the bathroom (either more urgently or more frequently).

But that's actually a good thing. Instead of having a whole bunch of carbs and sugars that pass around and create fat in your body, you can let the fiber pass right through you.

Try eating more foods that have fiber in them (or take a fiber drink or supplement). Here's some to get you started: Apples, grapefruit, raspberries, avocados, sweet corn, kale, bran cereal, oats, black beans, mixed nuts, seeds (flax seeds are the best), beans (kidney beans are the best), and brown rice.

81

EATING HEALTHY SNACKS

You know about portion control and learned that eating smaller snacks more frequently is better than eating large meals.

But you can't just claim cookies and ice cream as your 'small portioned' snack during the day. In order to truly get the benefit out of snacking or grazing as some call it, you should start thinking about just how healthy those snacks are.

You might think something like crackers or goldfish (the cheese cracker snack) are simple non-fatty snacks. Wrong. Eat enough of those and you'll gain weight in just a couple days.

Fresh fruit is good. Same with veggies. If you are going for crackers, go for the ones high in fiber - try wheat thins or something similar. But again, even the healthy snacks can cause you to gain weight if you eat a big enough portion. So, control your portions and eat healthy snacks and you'll be fine throughout the day.

82

AVOIDING FAD DIETS

You know those diets you see on TV or maybe a sales page on the internet that have those wacky promises?

These are the fad diets, and you should stay away from them as much as possible.

Whenever you see or hear that you "don't have to do any work" or it's just "one easy payment away" from success, you know it's a scam. Any time someone can make some money from a new workout routine or weight loss diet or even worse the "magic pills", they'll do it. They'll make the product, they'll get the celebrity endorsement, they'll pay for it all. And they'll gladly take your money any way they can, whether or not you get results.

Why isn't there ONE diet that has worked for 100+ years? It's because there are so many options for losing weight, every new technique seems like something no one has thought of before, yet it's usually the same types of things every time.

These fad diets come and go like clockwork, each cashing in on a new (or sometimes same) set of bodies.

Just because "Cindy from Ohio" lost 50 pounds using "Potion Z" doesn't mean you or anyone else will get the same if any results (as it always says in the fine print, just big enough to avoid the lawyers).

You'll only be going in circles with these false promises. Stick to the little things, stick to what actually works. Stick with natural weight loss, and you'll be happy with your results.

83

WISE RESTAURANT EATING

Besides portion controlling your food at restaurants, there are also a few more things you can do to help lose weight - we'll call this "wise restaurant eating".

I'm sure you'll be able to think of your own after these initial ideas, but take into consideration these 3 ideas for eating wisely at restaurants to lose weight:

1. Ask the waiter/waitress for the healthiest option(s). Most restaurants have a healthy eating section, or even something about the calories in certain dishes. And if not, you can always ask your waiter or waitress and they will be happy to tell you their healthiest choices to choose from.

2. Eat a salad instead of an appetizer. Don't go for the boneless wings, or the garlic bread, or the jalapeno poppers. Go for the salad, add chicken if you want. Salad means veggies, and the most delicious veggies for me has always been salad.

3. Share your food! Don't hog everything, share around. You should have already portioned your dinner at the start, so even if your friends or family eat half of your meal, you really have a whole other portion ready to eat! Let your friends and family take some weight off your hands. If you are still hungry, have some more. If you are full, be happy at the fact that you didn't consume more weight than you needed.

84

THE RULE OF 1

This is a great rule to follow, it's called the rule of 1.

Remember when we talked about rewarding yourself for accomplishing your weight loss goals? You learned that you shouldn't always reward yourself with food rewards to avoid putting back on unwanted weight after working so hard to lose it.

Sometimes, it's nice to have a treat every once in awhile. If you are going to reward yourself with treats, follow the rule of 1 and limit yourself to one food treat per day.

Maybe you reward yourself with a small cookie when you do 3 physical tasks during the day. You could have one glass of soda if you really really like it, but only after you've worked out for at least an hour.

When you limit yourself to 1 food treat per day, you build up willpower as well as treat yourself, making accomplishing tasks both fun and easy.

85

AFTER 8 IS TOO LATE

I wanted to end the food and diet section with my favorite saying for weight loss - "After 8 is too late!".

When you eat right before you go to sleep, the food is harder to digest, and basically sits in your stomach for longer than it should. And as you learned earlier, eating before bed stretches out your stomach while you sleep, making you even hungrier the next morning.

So, what a lot of us fitness freaks are following is the simple rhyme, "after 8 is too late". Of course this meaning after 8:00PM is too late to eat any type of food, even if it is healthy.

Make sure you are healthy snacking during the day. Eat dinner earlier. Once 8:00PM comes around, you know that you are not to eat anything else for the rest of the night.

If you can stick to this rhyme and rule, it will greatly increase your chance at losing weight faster. You are cutting out a chunk of your day where you won't eat, and you are making your stomach NOT stretch the next day, avoiding even more food consumption. You will also feel better the next morning when you wake up, giving you more energy to lose more weight while doing the things you want to do during the day.

FITNESS, EXERCISE AND WORKOUT

Congratulations, you've made it to the fifth and final section of the book - fitness exercise and workout.

The planning and thinking and feeling was a good start. Learning how to motivate yourself was very important. Learning about easy dieting was fun and simple.

Now it's time for the bread and butter of weight loss - EXERCISE. Some people never exercise and lose the weight simply by eating better and working on their daily routines. However, even for them, exercise and fitness can be that last piece of the puzzle that sheds the pounds.

Enjoy section 5, and take notes on the simple yet important fitness and exercise tips that will help you lose the weight and keep it off for good.

86

WARM UP AND STRETCH

Exercising and working out starts with a simple warm up and/or stretch.

Trust me, especially if you haven't exercised in awhile, STRETCH. By stretching your muscles, you avoid unnecessary muscle pain and soreness later on. You will experience some soreness from the exercises (which is good), but you don't want to feel in pain every day, so start by stretching.

After stretching, do some quick warm ups to get your body moving. This can be walking around the block, or even walking in place. You could do some high knees or butt-kicker leg exercises. You can swing your arms around from side to side to get the blood flowing.

Stretching and warming up is just another way to prepare for exercising and working out, and generally just helps and eases your way into weight loss exercises and workouts.

87

GET A HEART RATE MONITOR

Go get a heart rate monitor, they aren't expensive at all!

Knowing your heart rate (especially while doing any physical activity like exercising or working out) is important, because you can see how far you are pushing yourself, and just how much further you can go.

Monitoring your heart rate is an easy way to see if you are staying healthy while exercising, as well as to see if any problems occur (in which you should seek immediate medical attention). If you are doing a medium workout and your heart rate skyrockets up to 170+, or at dangerous levels above 200, your heart rate monitor can save your life.

Besides being able to save your life (before it needs saving), your heart rate monitor can also push yourself to new limits by showing you when you can work out harder. One or more workout or exercise routines might feel exhausting, but seeing a lower heart rate allows you to regroup and tell yourself that you can push yourself harder.

88

STAY FLEXIBLE

When you want to lose weight, it's best to stay flexible. And yes, that means a lot of stretching.

People with excess body weight have much more fat than muscle, and one's muscles might have gotten very tight without a lot of varied movement over time.

When your muscles are tight and you haven't stretched much or often enough, you will get the bad soreness instead of good soreness. You can hurt yourself or have muscle pain when working out. You won't feel the full burn or get the full effect or importance of each exercise routine.

Stretch as often as possible. Get one of those workout elastic bands if you need to, and stretch your arms, legs, all the different muscles - triceps, biceps, forearms, shoulders, chest, hamstrings, calves, and all the other little muscles in between.

The more flexible you are, the easier it is to exercise and work out. And not only does it make it easier, it also allows you to get everything you can out of your workouts. Just being able to safely and easily pull a weight or run at a faster pace for a few minutes gets you that much closer to your overall weight loss goal.

89

START SLOW AND SIMPLE

Slow and steady wins the race.

If you are feeling overwhelmed, or working out and doing physical activities isn't really your thing (at least yet), start out slow and simple.

There are 2 ways you can do this really:

#1 - Start with simpler workout routines. Instead of 10 or 20 pound dumbells, use the elastic bands or small 2 pound weights, and work your way up. If you have weak legs and can't even lift the lowest amount, start with just the weight of your legs. When people have surgery and have to re-learn how to work their legs, they don't start with weights. They start with the weight of their own legs and body (less than that even), and slowly work their way up to the more involved workouts.

#2 - Start at a slower pace. Instead of just going for the easy workouts, try a more difficult workout or a workout machine you aren't as comfortable with. But instead of doing lots of repetitions, do some slow reps to start. You might only be able to do 1 or 2 full reps, and that's okay. Next time you'll do 3, soon you'll do 5, eventually 10. Then, you can move up a weight, and do 2, 3, 5, 10, and so on.

Don't feel like you have to use weights right away or do the same routines as others or pick a high speed on the treadmill or bike at first. Do what you are physically able to, and push yourself without beating yourself to the ground. Start slow so that you can continue to move up, move forward, and it will get easier each and every time you exercise.

90

LEAST FAVORITE ROUTINES

This tip is for when you have the hang of the simpler workout routines or exercises at slower paces.

You can't do the same routine over and over again for the rest of your life. Change things up, add new machines, new exercises, varied cardio.

One technique that I use whenever I go to the gym is start on my least favorite machine. It's the deadweight hamstring leg lifts that I'm not a big fan of. However, I know I need to strengthen my hamstrings and lose a bit of the flub as I call it - so I do the damn workout.

Better yet, I do it first. I start with my least favorite routine. Why? Because as soon as I'm finished with that first few minutes of my full session, I feel as if everything else I'll do the entire workout will always be easier than what I started with.

It does take some willpower to get that first decision going to start with your least favorite routine (which is why this is only recommended once you have the basics down), but once you get going you'll feel so great the rest of the workout.

91

BUILDING YOUR CORE

Building? I thought we were losing!?

We are, but right now we're talking about your core.

Your core is the group of muscles that surrounds your stomache and lower back area. It is your lower back muscles, your abdomen, and all the other muscles in between. I don't have a list of every muscle in "the core". The core is just something I refer to as the general middle group of muscles in your abdomen/lower back area.

The reason you want to build your core is because it can provide you with so much more power in any workout. When I wasn't working on my core but still working out, there were times where I'd drop the weights or I wouldn't be able to hold my arms up, as if I could hold the weight, but it was still bringing my entire body to the floor.

When I started to build my core muscles, I had that extra push to get through more repetitions. I could feel running get easier, as if I had this little band of muscles that helped move the rest of my body parts.

You can work on your core very easily. Stand straight up. Now keeping everything below your hips still, move the upper part of your body from left to right slowly 10 times back and forth. Now do it front to back (without moving your bottom half of your body!). Do you feel the burn in your abs, your sides, and your lower back?

Any exercises or workouts where you can feel the burn in these muscle groups is "working out your core". Start to build your core and do muscle exercises that work it out, and you'll find your workouts getting easier all the time. And on top of that, you will be shedding loads of belly fat weight off of you. You'll be building your core and thinning your stomach at the same time, giving you a nice double effect to your workout.

92

WALK, WALK, WALK...

You don't even have to run after reading this tip..

Come on, walking isn't tough, it's just one foot in front of the other. If 2 year olds can do it, so can you.

You don't have to drive to the gym, walk in, get on the treadmill, and track yourself while you walk for 1 or 2 or 3 miles. You don't even have to make your walk the main event. But just simply walking around more can help you lose weight.

Think about how often you are just sitting around doing nothing. Try doing things around the house that require you to stand, walk around a little. If there is a park or theater or pool or store nearby, take a nice stroll there instead of driving.

The more you walk, the easier it is to lose weight. It won't happen overnight or even on it's own, but when included with other weight loss strategies, it can give you another one of those little extra helpful pushes.

93

PEDOMETER TRACKING

How many steps did you take today?

The reason I wanted to give this tip it's own little chapter is because of how important it is, especially for most of us who get irritated when we can't directly track our progress.

When I started walking more, I wasn't seeing the weight drop. I didn't feel like I was getting any thinner. Even though I knew I was walking and feeling a little better day by day, I still hated the fact that I couldn't directly see the progress I was making.

UNTIL.... I got a pedometer, which is basically just a little digital tracker tool that tracks how many steps you take (and some can track a lot more, like how many miles you've walked, etc.). They make handheld pedometers, ones built straight into your walking/running shoes, ones that hook on to your pants or belt loop.

Wow, did my mindset change when I found out I was walking 5,000 - 10,000 steps each day! And I'm sure it was probably just me feeling better about my walking, but I started to notice my legs and tummy getting thinner, I noticed the little hanging fat on my cheeks disappear.

This is another visual and mental cue that you can use to show yourself that you are indeed making progress at all times. 1,000 steps? 3,000? You'll be surprised at just how much and how far you can walk in a day, and you'll know that you are always moving forward when you take a glance at your pedometer. These things are inexpensive, so go buy one right now and start using it.

94

Sign Up For A Race

I know that the last thing any overweight person wants to do is sign up for a race.

Remember my brother who bought the smaller pants and shirts and started to lose weight? It's because he was preparing himself (both his mind and body) for his own future.

Same goes with signing up for a race. It doesn't need to be a 26 mile marathon, or even a half marathon. It can be as little as a mile or 2 race that "normal humans" can race in.

The point is to sign up for the race and make yourself accountable for losing the weight, getting as much in shape as you can, drinking more water, practicing your walking and jogging. With no race or event ahead, there's no true timeline of tasks and events that NEED to occur before anything, you are able to choose when and where and how often you work on losing weight.

When the big race is in 2 or 3 months, your body and mind will WANT to prepare yourself for what is to come. And no matter how you do in the race, the real win is you racing in general. Sign up for a walk or jog or running race today, sign up for one that is happening a few months in advance. Promise yourself that you will attend the race no matter what, and you'll be more motivated than ever to get into better shape.

And when the race is over, it doesn't matter what your time was or what place you got. Mark down your time, and then sign up for another race. Now your goal isn't to just get to the race and run it it, but actually beat your previous time.

95

FAVORITE WORKOUT MUSIC

We all have our favorite music that gets us pumped up, gets us moving, thinking, that music that brings feeling and emotion inside of us.

I would be bored to death without my workout music. For me, I like the fast paced dance music, and maybe sometimes some rock - anything that's going to get my blood flowing and my body moving.

Get an mp3 player, a CD player, a boombox, a radio, something that can play music. If you work out at the gym, get some headphones. If you are at home or not in a public place, you can use speakers and crank up the volume!

You can use music in a few different ways while working out. You can use it to get you over the first hump or the first exercise. You can use the beats in the song as your reps on the weights or as your footsteps on the treadmill. You can use your favorite music to inspire you. Your favorite music can bring you emotions and feelings that make you happy, which can make your workout easier and actually fun.

If you are in a slump, put on some music. Do a little dance if you want. Get in the zone, and get going on your workout.

96

OUTDOOR
EXERCISE ROUTINES

Need some fresh air? Sometimes you've just got to get out of the house, out of the gym.

The great outdoors. There is more fresh air outside. There are more natural sounds, more peace (at times), more excitement and energy.

There's so much outside, so get out and enjoy it during your next exercise routine.

It's okay if you don't want to go to the public park - try this first in your backyard. Do some leg exercises, get a jump rope, stretch your arms and legs on a tree or bench. Run in place, use some elastic exercise bands.

Going outside changes up the pace a little, changes your environment. Sometimes we get bored inside, sometimes we get cramped, constricted. And sometimes all we need is a little change of surroundings, and instantly we are able to find a new motivation or new view on the task at hand - this time being outdoor exercise.

97

BUILDING MUSCLE

You're trying to lose weight, so you might be confused as to why we want you to GAIN muscle (therefore gaining more weight).

First take a thought at this: When you walk, you aren't just losing weight, you're gaining muscle (at a slower pace) in all of your muscles that are used as you walk - this includes legs, arms, core, everything really.

Building muscle actually helps you lose fat, since building muscle burns calories.

And when we're really talking about losing weight, we are talking about losing FAT. There are 200 pound guys full of big muscle, and there are 150 pound women who are skinny with strong tight muscles. You can weigh a lot and have literally 1% fat in your body only.

Start with some simple dumbell exercises, and build up from there. Do more repetitions, add some weight. Go to the gym and try the machines - get your workout buddy in there with you!

When you feel the burn in your muscles and the good soreness it leaves after, you'll know that you are becoming stronger and burning fat at the same time. Just make sure you aren't working out your muscles hard every single day - they need time to rest! When you "build muscle", you are actually tearing it down during the initial workout, and then it recovers over the next few days/weeks and builds muscle during this time (and burns fat of course).

98

EXERCISE EXPLORING

It's time to have some fitness fun!

After some time of doing the same exercises, same machines, same workouts all the time, you may begin to feel bored and unmotivated before working out.

But what you need to realize is - It is not the weight loss that becomes not fun or boring, it is the way in which you lose the weight that becomes not fun or boring.

All you have to do in order to get back in the groove is explore some new exercises and workout routines! Take the following tips, write them down, and use them when your workout routine isn't living up to your standards:

1. Exploring brand new exercises. Stop doing the same situps and pushups - try something new. There are hundreds of different ways to get the same situp/crunch feeling. You can work out your arms in even more ways. As long as you feel the burn, the sweat, and the workout, anything can be exercise.

2. Have fun (instead of) exercise. I put "instead of" in parentheses because you're actually going to be exercising, but it doesn't seem like it. Think about things you can do during the day that are fun, but also get you sweating or moving around or lifting something. Walk the dog, take a swim, play a physical game like tag or hide and seek. If you don't like games but still like fun, why don't you walk around the mall? Maybe go to the beach? You can have the most fun-filled life, be happy, and exercise all day long.

3. Check out the world wide web. Go ahead, type in "exercise" on YouTube or Google. You'll find millions of results (billions? wow). Every day, people are coming out with new videos and articles regarding new and fun workout routines, exercises, as well as the motivation that most of us need to get going. Spend a good 30 minutes to an hour right now searching around

online, and you'll find some new fun routines for you to implement.

The point of exploring new exercises is so you never get bored. You want to continue moving forward towards your weight loss goals, and any little thing you can do during the day to add to your weight loss will help you that much more.

99

AVOIDING TALKATIVE TANYA

Talkative Tanya, Tammy, Thomas - they should be avoided at all costs.

This is a tip for all of you gym-goers or people who exercise with or around others in a public (or even private) setting.

Have you ever gone to the gym only to be bombarded by your "friend" who would rather gossip or talk to you about possibly interesting stuff instead of working out and making themselves better?

If everytime you go to the gym you are being talked to almost all workout-long, you should find another gym. Or, you can put on headphones and avoid those people alltogether. The reason you want to avoid these people is because although they are probably not trying to disrupt you or distract you, they are still causing you to lose weight SLOWER and HARDER.

The more you talk while you work out, the more energy you are wasting on words and the less energy you are using to lose weight. You can talk to your friend or 2 at the gym, but while you are working out, don't talk to anyone unless it is a question to your trainer or workout buddy.

Your workout time is worth gold to your weight loss journey, so don't mess it up. Just stay on your path and do work.

BONUS

STEPS TO TAKE IMMEDIATELY FOR BEST RESULTS

Congratulations!

You've finished the book, bringing you one step closer on your weight loss journey. I wanted to give you a little additional info to help lead you in the right direction so you can get started immediately and implement what you just learned into your life.

There were 99 tips in this book, but there's no way you'll be able to follow every single one 100% every day all day all the time...

BUT - What I recommend is that you go back through this book (faster this time since you've read it once already) and choose your favorite tips. Besides your favorites, choose the ones that you actually know you will be able to accomplish. Maybe you just can't cut out soda or alcohol, but you CAN hit the gym, drink more water and eat more foods that are high in fiber.

Your weight loss journey is different than mine, in fact everyone's weight loss happens at least a little bit differently. There's absolutely no way 2 people could follow the same exact program, mindset changes, workout routines, and diet EXACTLY the same. Sure we can both eat more fiber, but the fiber you choose will be different than mine.

It is important to understand this, because many people think they need an exact plan, or that there is a 100% proven science to losing an exact amount of weight that works for 100% of the people on the planet. It just doesn't work that way.

For instance, here's an example of how you might group together your favorite tips into your own weight loss plan:

- First, I can definitely get my mindset in the right place, and do the basic mind shifts, motivation tactics, envisioning, journaling, and planning. I might not be able to get to bed as early as I should, but I can drink lemon water as soon as I wake up. I don't like apples or bananas, but I'm fine with eating oatmeal which is high in fiber and good for me. I can get a heart rate monitor and a pedometer, I'm fine with walking. I won't sign up for a race, but I'll motivate myself in the gym with a new playlist I made. I can also avoid talkative people in the gym, in fact I hate talking to people in the gym.

While that might be the part of one person's plan, another can be completely different and still yield weight loss results, for instance:

- I'll do my best to motivate myself. I'll sign myself up for a race. I'll try to do all the diet stuff, but it's hard for me to work out and exercise as much as I need to. I can go to bed earlier, especially if it will help me lose weight. I can stretch every morning, and instead of lemon water I might have a green tea in the morning. I can try to focus on my meal so I know when I'm full - I'll also take the 2 minute meal break every time. It's hard to keep track of protein/carbs/fat sources, but I can definitely remove the skin from the chicken. I don't like skimmed milk, but I'll stay away from fast food and processed food.

Do you see how this works?

Even if it isn't a complete plan, it is important that you take at least 30 minutes (even up to a couple hours) to put together a general plan and just get started on something. It all starts with the little steps, the thoughts, the mind shifts. The actions that you take today will benefit you and will ensure the future self you want to be.

Trust me, once you get going on your weight loss journey from the plan you make right now, it will keep getting easier. You'll follow 5 of these tips immediately, and lose some pounds in a week or two. Then you'll say, "Wow, that seemed easier than I thought. Let's try some more!". Then you'll add in some more on top of what you are already doing, and you'll lose even more weight. By the time you have this weight loss thing down, you'll have a complete grasp on things, probably enough to share how you did it with your friends and family.

Who knows, maybe you'll inspire someone else to do something similar to what you did. Maybe you'll inspire them just in time. Maybe you'll save someone's life. Maybe you'll save 100 lives.

You never know until you do it, so why not start right now?

I'm not going to wish you luck, because luck isn't what's needed. What's needed, is action.

Amy Culderson and Mike Shaw

Thanks For Reading!

Thank you so much for reading this book. We had a lot of fun writing it, and are pumped to hear about how these tips work out for you and your weight loss journey.

I honestly want to hear from you, and I'm not talking about a month from now when you've lost your first few pounds (or more). I'm talking about right NOW. Take a quick click over to the book info page for Lose The Weight: 99 Weight Loss Tips, and tell me you are going to try these tips. Tell me you have a plan, tell the WORLD you have a plan. There's no better way to start your journey than by telling the world that you are here, you are ready, and you have started your journey.

We all start somewhere. No one is ever born with complete knowledge and understanding of losing weight, or anything for that matter. The point is that you have started, and you will keep going forward as the weight keeps going down.

Leave us a review right now, and I'll read it. Then I'll think of you and send positive energy your way. Truthfully, I will.

Thank you again, I truly hope you enjoyed this book and these tips, NOW GET STARTED!

www.ingramcontent.com/pod-product-compliance
Lightning Source LLC
Chambersburg PA
CBHW070537290526
45790CB00002B/536